METABOLIC RESET DIET

COOKBOOK FOR ENDOMORPH

Nutritional guide with a 28-day meal plan to Lose Weight Naturally and balance Hormones with over 70 tasty recipes

Dr. JANE THORNTHWAITE

TABLE OF CONTENTS

Chapter 1

Introduction

Understanding the Endomorph Body Type

The endomorph body type is one of the three categories in the somatotype classification system, which describes human bodies based on their propensity towards certain physical and metabolic characteristics. Endomorphs are often distinguished by their rounder, more voluptuous physique, characterized by a higher proportion of body fat, a tendency to gain weight easily, and a struggle with losing it. Unlike ectomorphs, who are lean and find it hard to gain weight, or mesomorphs, who are muscular and can easily gain or lose weight, endomorphs have a specific set of challenges and strengths related to their body composition and metabolism.

Endomorphs often experience a slower metabolic rate compared to their ectomorphic and mesomorphic counterparts, who are characterized by leaner frames and more muscular builds, respectively. This slower metabolism signifies a more efficient fat storage system, which, while beneficial in times of scarcity, poses challenges in the modern world where food is abundant and often highly processed.

The metabolic intricacies of the endomorph body type extend into how it processes macronutrients, particularly carbohydrates. Insulin sensitivity can lead to difficulties in managing blood sugar levels, influencing not only weight gain but also energy fluctuations throughout the day. This sensitivity necessitates a mindful approach to diet, one that balances macronutrients in a way that supports metabolic health and promotes a stable energy supply.

Understanding and embracing the endomorph body type is not merely about accepting a biological predisposition but about recognizing the unique potential for transformation that lies within. It's about navigating the journey of health and fitness with knowledge and intention, tailoring nutrition and exercise to harness the strengths of the endomorph body type while mitigating its challenges. This journey is deeply personal, reflecting not just a quest for physical health but a commitment to holistic well-being.

Principles of the Metabolic Reset Diet

The Metabolic Reset Diet is centered on the concept of reinvigorating and optimizing the body's metabolic processes to enhance weight loss, improve energy levels, and foster overall health and wellness. This dietary approach is grounded in understanding how various foods and lifestyle choices can influence metabolism—the body's engine for burning calories and converting food to energy. Unlike traditional diets that often focus on strict calorie restriction or eliminating entire food groups, the Metabolic Reset Diet aims to achieve a balanced and sustainable way of eating that supports the body's natural ability to regulate weight and health.

At the heart of the Metabolic Reset Diet is the recognition of the body's remarkable ability to adapt and change in response to nutritional and lifestyle inputs. This diet encourages a holistic approach to eating and living, acknowledging that factors such as sleep quality, stress levels, and physical activity all play integral roles in metabolic health. The diet emphasizes the importance of consuming whole, nutrient-dense foods that provide the body with the energy and nutrients it needs to function optimally, without overloading it with empty calories that can disrupt metabolic balance.

One of the foundational principles of the Metabolic Reset Diet is the focus on improving insulin sensitivity and managing blood sugar levels. By selecting foods that have a minimal impact on blood sugar spikes, individuals can maintain steadier energy levels throughout the day, reduce cravings, and minimize the risk of storing excess calories as fat. This approach often involves moderating carbohydrate intake, prioritizing complex carbs that are high in fiber, and balancing them with adequate protein and healthy fats to stabilize blood sugar and enhance satiety.

How This Cookbook Can Help

This cookbook is designed as a transformative tool for individuals aiming to navigate the unique challenges of the endomorph body type, particularly in resetting their metabolism to achieve a more balanced and healthy lifestyle. At its core, it recognizes the critical role that diet plays not only in weight management but also in influencing metabolic efficiency, energy levels, and overall well-being. By providing a carefully curated selection of recipes that align with the principles of the Metabolic Reset Diet, this cookbook serves as a practical guide to making dietary choices that are conducive to the needs of endomorphs.

This approach helps stabilize blood sugar levels, reduce cravings, and promote a feeling of fullness, thereby avoiding the common pitfalls of overeating or relying on processed foods.

Moreover, this cookbook emphasizes the importance of meal variety and flavor, debunking the myth that healthy eating for metabolic reset has to be monotonous or bland. It introduces creative ways to enjoy fruits, vegetables, lean proteins, and healthy fats, making it easier to adhere to a metabolic-friendly diet without feeling deprived. Each recipe is accompanied by clear nutritional information, serving suggestions, and tips for meal prepping, making it accessible for both novices and seasoned cooks.

Chapter 2

Fundamentals of Nutrition for Endomorphs

Macronutrient Ratios and Choices

For individuals with the endomorph body type, managing macronutrient ratios is pivotal in optimizing metabolism, supporting weight management, and fostering overall health. The key macronutrients—proteins, carbohydrates, and fats—must be balanced in a way that aligns with the endomorph's slower metabolic rate and potential insulin sensitivity. This balance helps in mitigating fat storage and promoting the use of stored fat as energy, thereby aiding in weight loss and the maintenance of lean muscle mass.

Protein is essential for endomorphs as it has a high thermogenic effect, meaning it requires more energy for digestion, absorption, and assimilation than carbohydrates and fats. A diet rich in lean proteins from sources such as poultry, fish, legumes, and low-fat dairy products can enhance satiety, reduce cravings, and support muscle repair and growth. Incorporating adequate protein in every meal is crucial for stimulating metabolism and preserving muscle mass while losing weight.

Carbohydrates should be selected carefully, favoring complex carbohydrates with a low glycemic index (GI) such as whole grains, vegetables, and certain fruits. These carbs are digested more slowly, providing a gradual release of energy and maintaining stable blood sugar levels, which is vital for controlling appetite and minimizing fat storage.

Fats, particularly those from healthy sources like avocados, nuts, seeds, and olive oil, play a vital role in hormone production and satiety. Incorporating moderate amounts of healthy fats can enhance flavor, increase nutrient absorption, and prevent overeating.

For endomorphs, a general macronutrient ratio that often proves effective is a higher proportion of protein, a moderate amount of fat, and a lower intake of carbohydrates. However, individual needs can vary, and adjustments might be necessary based on personal health goals, activity levels, and metabolic responses.

Importance of Fiber and Whole Foods

In the journey towards metabolic optimization and weight management, especially for endomorphs, the importance of fiber and whole foods cannot be overstated. Incorporating a diet rich in fiber and whole foods plays a critical role in enhancing digestive health, regulating blood sugar levels, and supporting sustainable weight loss.

Fiber, a vital nutrient found in plant-based foods, offers multiple benefits for metabolic health. It aids in digestion, helps to keep the gastrointestinal tract functioning smoothly, and promotes a feeling of fullness, which can prevent overeating and assist in weight control. By slowing down the absorption of sugar into the bloodstream, high-fiber foods also help in managing insulin sensitivity—a common concern for endomorphs. This regulation of blood sugar levels is crucial for avoiding spikes and crashes that can lead to increased hunger and fat storage.

Whole foods, such as vegetables, fruits, whole grains, legumes, nuts, and seeds, are naturally rich in fiber and essential nutrients. Unlike processed foods, which often contain added sugars, unhealthy fats, and artificial ingredients, whole foods provide the body with a synergy of vitamins, minerals, and antioxidants needed for optimal health. These nutrient-dense foods support metabolic functions, enhance energy levels, and contribute to the body's overall well-being.

For endomorphs, focusing on a diet dominated by fiber-rich whole foods can significantly impact their metabolic reset journey. It encourages a holistic approach to eating that not only addresses weight management but also promotes a healthier, more balanced lifestyle. By making these nutrient-packed foods the cornerstone of their diet, endomorphs can navigate the challenges of their body type more effectively, paving the way for improved metabolic health and sustainable weight management.

Managing Carbohydrate Intake

For individuals with the endomorph body type, managing carbohydrate intake is a crucial aspect of maintaining a healthy metabolism and facilitating weight loss. Endomorphs tend to have a slower metabolic rate and may be more sensitive to insulin, a hormone that regulates blood sugar levels. This sensitivity can lead to an increased likelihood of storing excess carbohydrates as fat, rather than using them for energy. Therefore, careful management of carbohydrate intake is essential to avoid unwanted weight gain and support metabolic health.

Choosing the right types of carbohydrates is key. It is beneficial for endomorphs to focus on consuming low-glycemic index (GI) carbohydrates that are digested and absorbed slowly, helping to maintain stable blood sugar levels and reduce insulin spikes. Foods such as whole grains, legumes, vegetables, and some fruits are excellent choices because they provide sustained energy, are rich in nutrients, and contribute to a feeling of fullness, which can help control appetite.

Portion control is another important factor in managing carbohydrate intake. Even healthy carbohydrates can contribute to weight gain if consumed in large quantities. Endomorphs should moderate their carbohydrate portions, making sure they complement their diet with adequate protein and healthy fats to balance the overall macronutrient profile.

Timing of carbohydrate consumption can also play a role in metabolic efficiency. Consuming carbohydrates around physical activity, for example, can ensure that the sugars are used for energy rather than stored as fat. This strategy can be particularly effective for endomorphs looking to improve their body composition and enhance their metabolic rate.

Chapter 3

28-day Meal plan for metabolic reset

Week 1

Day 1:

- **Breakfast:** Avocado Toast with Poached Egg
- **Snack:** Greek Yogurt with Berries
- **Lunch:** Grilled Chicken Salad with Balsamic Vinaigrette
- **Snack:** Carrot Sticks with Hummus
- **Dinner:** Baked Salmon with Roasted Vegetables
- **Dessert:** Chia Seed Pudding

Day 2:

- **Breakfast:** Green Smoothie
- **Snack:** Apple Slices with Almond Butter
- **Lunch:** Quinoa Salad with Chickpeas and Veggies

- **Snack:** Mixed Nuts
- **Dinner:** Turkey Meatballs with Zucchini Noodles
- **Dessert:** Mixed Berry Parfait

Day 3:

- **Breakfast:** Oatmeal with Banana Slices and Almonds
- **Snack:** Cottage Cheese with Pineapple Chunks
- **Lunch:** Lentil Soup with Whole Grain Bread
- **Snack:** Celery Sticks with Peanut Butter
- **Dinner:** Stir-fried tofu with Broccoli and Brown Rice
- **Dessert:** Dark Chocolate Covered Strawberries

Day 4:

- **Breakfast:** Scrambled Eggs with Spinach and Tomatoes

- **Snack:** Sliced Cucumber with Hummus
- **Lunch:** Quinoa Stuffed Bell Peppers
- **Snack:** Greek Yogurt with Granola
- **Dinner:** Grilled Shrimp with Quinoa and Asparagus
- **Dessert:** Banana "Nice" Cream

Day 5:

- **Breakfast:** Whole Grain Pancakes with Berries and Greek Yogurt
- **Snack:** Almonds and Dried Apricots
- **Lunch:** Chicken Caesar Salad Wrap
- **Snack:** Rice Cakes with Cottage Cheese and Tomato Slices
- **Dinner:** Baked Cod with Roasted Sweet Potatoes and Green Beans
- **Dessert:** Baked Apple with Cinnamon

Day 6:

- **Breakfast:** Breakfast Burrito with Whole Wheat Tortilla, Scrambled Eggs, Black Beans, and Salsa
- **Snack:** Bell Pepper Strips with Hummus
- **Lunch:** Quinoa and Black Bean Salad
- **Snack:** Cottage Cheese with Peach Slices
- **Dinner:** Vegetable Stir-Fry with Tofu and Brown Rice
- **Dessert:** Mango Coconut Chia Pudding

Day 7:

- **Breakfast:** Overnight Oats with Mixed Berries and Almond Milk
- **Snack:** Hard-boiled Egg
- **Lunch:** Turkey and Avocado Wrap with Whole Wheat Tortilla
- **Snack:** Edamame

- **Dinner:** Grilled Chicken Breast with Steamed Broccoli and Quinoa
- **Dessert:** Aloe Vera Refresh Drink

Week 2

Day 8:

- **Breakfast:** Spinach and Feta Omelette with Whole Grain Toast
- **Snack:** Cottage Cheese with Pineapple Chunks
- **Lunch:** Mediterranean Chickpea Salad
- **Snack:** Mixed Nuts
- **Dinner:** Grilled Vegetable and Chicken Skewers with Quinoa
- **Dessert:** Cinnamon Almond Milk Warmer

Day 9:

- **Breakfast:** Blueberry Banana Smoothie

- **Snack:** Apple Slices with Almond Butter
- **Lunch:** Lentil and Vegetable Stir-Fry
- **Snack:** Carrot Sticks with Hummus
- **Dinner:** Baked Cod with Lemon Garlic Butter Sauce and Asparagus
- **Dessert:** Refreshing Watermelon Mint Juice

Day 10:

- **Breakfast:** Protein Pancakes with Greek Yogurt and Berries
- **Snack:** Mixed Berries with Cottage Cheese
- **Lunch:** Turkey and Veggie Wrap with Whole Wheat Tortilla
- **Snack:** Rice Cakes with Peanut Butter and Banana Slices
- **Dinner:** Grilled Salmon with Roasted Brussels Sprouts and Sweet Potatoes

- **Dessert:** Apple Cinnamon Quinoa Breakfast Bowl

Day 11:

- **Breakfast:** Veggie Breakfast Burrito with Scrambled Eggs and Avocado
- **Snack:** Celery Sticks with Hummus
- **Lunch:** Quinoa and Black Bean Stuffed Bell Peppers
- **Snack:** Greek Yogurt with Granola
- **Dinner:** Spaghetti Squash with Turkey Bolognese Sauce
- **Dessert:** Dark Chocolate Avocado Mousse

Day 12:

- **Breakfast:** Greek Yogurt Parfait with Mixed Berries and Granola
- **Snack:** Almonds and Dried Apricots
- **Lunch:** Chicken and Vegetable Stir-Fry with Brown Rice

- **Snack:** Bell Pepper Strips with Hummus
- **Dinner:** Baked Chicken Breast with Steamed Green Beans and Quinoa
- **Dessert:** Strawberry Banana Smoothie Bowl

Day 13:

- **Breakfast:** Whole Grain Waffles with Fresh Fruit and Greek Yogurt
- **Snack:** Hard-boiled Egg
- **Lunch:** Lentil Soup with Whole Grain Bread
- **Snack:** Cottage Cheese with Peach Slices
- **Dinner:** Grilled Shrimp Tacos with Cabbage Slaw and Avocado
- **Dessert:** Mango Coconut Chia Pudding

Day 14:

- **Breakfast:** Overnight Chia Seed Pudding with Mixed Berries
- **Snack:** Edamame
- **Lunch:** Quinoa Salad with Chickpeas, Cucumber, and Feta Cheese
- **Snack:** Carrot Sticks with Almond Butter
- **Dinner:** Turkey Meatballs with Zucchini Noodles and Marinara Sauce
- **Dessert:** Baked Apple with Cinnamon

Week 3

Day 15:

- **Breakfast:** Veggie Egg Muffins with Spinach, Bell Peppers, and Feta Cheese
- **Snack:** Greek Yogurt with Honey and Walnuts

- **Lunch:** Quinoa and Black Bean Burrito Bowl with Avocado and Salsa
- **Snack:** Sliced Cucumber with Hummus
- **Dinner:** Grilled Chicken Caesar Salad with Whole Grain Croutons
- **Dessert:** Berry Smoothie with Protein Powder

Day 16:

- **Breakfast:** Banana Oatmeal Pancakes with Maple Syrup
- **Snack:** Mixed Berries with Cottage Cheese
- **Lunch:** Lentil and Vegetable Curry with Brown Rice
- **Snack:** Rice Cakes with Almond Butter and Banana Slices
- **Dinner:** Baked Salmon with Roasted Asparagus and Quinoa

- **Dessert:** Chocolate Chia Seed Pudding

Day 17:

- **Breakfast:** Spinach and Mushroom Frittata with Whole Grain Toast
- **Snack:** Apple Slices with Peanut Butter
- **Lunch:** Turkey and Avocado Wrap with Lettuce and Tomato
- **Snack:** Carrot Sticks with Hummus
- **Dinner:** Grilled Veggie and Tofu Skewers with Brown Rice
- **Dessert:** Mixed Berry Parfait with Greek Yogurt

Day 18:

- **Breakfast:** Protein-Packed Smoothie Bowl with Almond Milk, Spinach, and Berries
- **Snack:** Hard-boiled Egg

- **Lunch:** Quinoa and Chickpea Salad with Mixed Greens and Lemon Vinaigrette
- **Snack:** Mixed Nuts and Dried Fruit
- **Dinner:** Baked Chicken Breast with Steamed Broccoli and Sweet Potato Mash
- **Dessert:** Greek Yogurt with Honey and Sliced Almonds

Day 19:

- **Breakfast:** Whole Grain French Toast with Fresh Fruit and Greek Yogurt
- **Snack:** Cottage Cheese with Pineapple Chunks
- **Lunch:** Lentil Soup with Whole Grain Bread
- **Snack:** Bell Pepper Strips with Hummus
- **Dinner:** Turkey Chili with Black Beans and Quinoa

- **Dessert:** Banana "Nice" Cream with Dark Chocolate Shavings

Day 20:

- **Breakfast:** Scrambled Eggs with Spinach, Tomato, and Feta Cheese
- **Snack:** Celery Sticks with Almond Butter
- **Lunch:** Quinoa and Black Bean Stuffed Peppers with Avocado Slices
- **Snack:** Greek Yogurt with Granola and Berries
- **Dinner:** Grilled Shrimp with Quinoa Pilaf and Steamed Vegetables
- **Dessert:** Mango Coconut Chia Pudding

Day 21:

- **Breakfast:** Overnight Oats with Chia Seeds, Almond Milk, and Mixed Berries
- **Snack:** Edamame

- **Lunch:** Chicken Caesar Salad Wrap with Whole Wheat Tortilla
- **Snack:** Rice Cakes with Cottage Cheese and Tomato Slices
- **Dinner:** Baked Cod with Lemon Herb Sauce and Roasted Brussels Sprouts
- **Dessert:** Aloe Vera Refresh Drink

Week 4

Day 22:

- **Breakfast:** Green Smoothie Bowl with Spinach, Banana, and Almond Butter
- **Snack:** Greek Yogurt with Honey and Walnuts
- **Lunch:** Quinoa Salad with Roasted Vegetables and Feta Cheese
- **Snack:** Carrot Sticks with Hummus
- **Dinner:** Grilled Chicken Breast with Quinoa Pilaf and Steamed Broccoli
- **Dessert:** Chocolate Avocado Mousse

Day 23:

- **Breakfast:** Veggie Breakfast Burrito with Scrambled Eggs, Black Beans, and Salsa
- **Snack:** Apple Slices with Peanut Butter
- **Lunch:** Lentil Soup with Whole Grain Bread
- **Snack:** Mixed Nuts and Dried Fruit
- **Dinner:** Baked Salmon with Garlic Herb Butter and Roasted Asparagus
- **Dessert:** Mixed Berry Smoothie with Protein Powder

Day 24:

- **Breakfast:** Whole Grain Pancakes with Maple Syrup and Fresh Fruit
- **Snack:** Cottage Cheese with Pineapple Chunks
- **Lunch:** Turkey and Avocado Wrap with Lettuce, Tomato, and Mustard

- **Snack:** Sliced Cucumber with Hummus
- **Dinner:** Grilled Veggie Stir-Fry with Tofu and Brown Rice
- **Dessert:** Chia Seed Pudding with Almond Milk and Berries

Day 25:

- **Breakfast:** Scrambled Eggs with Spinach, Mushrooms, and Feta Cheese
- **Snack:** Greek Yogurt with Granola and Mixed Berries
- **Lunch:** Quinoa and Black Bean Salad with Cucumber, Tomato, and Lime Vinaigrette
- **Snack:** Bell Pepper Strips with Hummus
- **Dinner:** Baked Chicken Thighs with Roasted Sweet Potatoes and Green Beans

- **Dessert:** Banana "Nice" Cream with Dark Chocolate Chips

Day 26:

- **Breakfast:** Blueberry Banana Protein Smoothie
- **Snack:** Hard-boiled Egg
- **Lunch:** Mediterranean Chickpea Salad with Mixed Greens and Lemon Vinaigrette
- **Snack:** Rice Cakes with Almond Butter and Banana Slices
- **Dinner:** Turkey Meatballs with Marinara Sauce and Zucchini Noodles
- **Dessert:** Coconut Mango Smoothie Bowl

Day 27:

- **Breakfast:** Overnight Oats with Almond Milk, Chia Seeds, and Mixed Berries

- **Snack:** Mixed Berries with Cottage Cheese
- **Lunch:** Lentil and Vegetable Stir-Fry with Brown Rice
- **Snack:** Carrot Sticks with Hummus
- **Dinner:** Grilled Shrimp Tacos with Cabbage Slaw and Avocado
- **Dessert:** Chocolate Covered Strawberries

Day 28:

- **Breakfast:** Veggie Egg Scramble with Spinach, Bell Peppers, and Onion
- **Snack:** Greek Yogurt with Honey and Walnuts
- **Lunch:** Quinoa Stuffed Bell Peppers with Black Beans, Corn, and Salsa
- **Snack:** Apple Slices with Almond Butter
- **Dinner:** Baked Cod with Tomato Basil Relish and Steamed Broccoli

- **Dessert:** Mixed Berry Parfait with Greek Yogurt and Granola

Chapter 4

Breakfast Recipes

Avocado Egg Bake

Ingredients:

- 2 avocados, halved and pitted
- 4 eggs
- Salt and pepper, to taste
- 1 tablespoon chopped chives

Instructions:

1. Preheat oven to 425°F (220°C).
2. Scoop out a bit of avocado to create space for the egg.
3. Place avocados on a baking dish and crack an egg into each avocado half. Season with salt and pepper.
4. Bake for 15-20 minutes or until the eggs are cooked to your liking.
5. Garnish with chives.

Nutritional Information:

- Calories: 300
- Protein: 10g
- Fat: 27g
- Carbs: 13g
- Fiber: 10g

Spinach and Feta Omelette

Ingredients:

- 3 eggs
- 1 cup spinach, chopped
- 1/4 cup feta cheese, crumbled
- 1 tablespoon olive oil
- Salt and pepper, to taste

Instructions:

1. Beat the eggs with salt and pepper.
2. Heat olive oil in a pan over medium heat, add spinach and cook until wilted.

3. Pour the eggs over the spinach and sprinkle feta cheese on top.

4. Cook until the eggs are set, fold the omelette in half, and serve.

Nutritional Information:

- Calories: 320
- Protein: 22g
- Fat: 24g
- Carbs: 4g
- Fiber: 1g

Chia and Berry Parfait

Ingredients:

- 3 tablespoons chia seeds
- 1 cup almond milk
- 1/2 teaspoon vanilla extract
- 1 cup mixed berries
- 1 tablespoon chopped nuts (optional)

Instructions:

1. Mix chia seeds, almond milk, and vanilla extract in a bowl. Let it sit for 15 minutes or until it becomes gel-like.
2. Layer chia pudding with mixed berries in a glass or jar.
3. Top with chopped nuts for added crunch.

Nutritional Information:

- Calories: 280
- Protein: 8g
- Fat: 15g
- Carbs: 30g
- Fiber: 14g

Protein Pancakes

Ingredients:

- 1 cup oats
- 1 banana
- 2 eggs

- 1/2 cup Greek yogurt
- 1 teaspoon vanilla extract
- 1/2 teaspoon cinnamon

Instructions:

1. Blend oats, bananas, eggs, Greek yogurt, vanilla extract, and cinnamon until smooth.
2. Heat a non-stick pan over medium heat and pour batter to form pancakes.
3. Cook until bubbles form on top, then flip and cook the other side.
4. Serve with a dollop of Greek yogurt and fresh berries.

Nutritional Information:

- Calories: 350
- Protein: 20g
- Fat: 7g
- Carbs: 55g
- Fiber: 8g

Smoked Salmon and Avocado Toast

Ingredients:

- 2 slices of whole-grain bread, toasted
- 1 avocado, mashed
- 4 oz smoked salmon
- 1 tablespoon lemon juice
- Salt and pepper, to taste
- Dill for garnish

Instructions:

1. Spread mashed avocado on toasted bread.
2. Top with smoked salmon, drizzle with lemon juice, and season with salt and pepper.
3. Garnish with dill before serving.

Nutritional Information:

- Calories: 400
- Protein: 23g
- Fat: 24g
- Carbs: 33g

- Fiber: 9g

Quinoa Breakfast Bowl

Ingredients:

- 1/2 cup cooked quinoa
- 1/4 cup almond milk
- 1 tablespoon almond butter
- 1/2 apple, chopped
- 1 tablespoon chia seeds
- Cinnamon, to taste

Instructions:

1. Warm the cooked quinoa and almond milk in a pot over medium heat.
2. Stir in the almond butter, chopped apple, and chia seeds until well combined.
3. Sprinkle with cinnamon and serve warm.

Nutritional Information:

- Calories: 350
- Protein: 10g
- Fat: 15g
- Carbs: 45g
- Fiber: 8g

Cottage Cheese and Peach Breakfast

Ingredients:

- 1 cup cottage cheese
- 1 peach, sliced
- 1 tablespoon flaxseeds
- Honey (optional)

Instructions:

1. Place cottage cheese in a bowl.
2. Top with sliced peach and sprinkle with flaxseeds.
3. Drizzle with honey if desired.

Nutritional Information:

- Calories: 220

- Protein: 28g

- Fat: 5g

- Carbs: 18g

- Fiber: 3g

Green Smoothie Bowl

Ingredients:

- 1 banana

- 1/2 cup spinach

- 1/4 avocado

- 1/2 cup almond milk

- 1 tablespoon protein powder

- Toppings: sliced fruits, nuts, seeds

Instructions:

1. Blend banana, spinach, avocado, almond milk, and protein powder until smooth.

2. Pour into a bowl and add your favorite toppings.

Nutritional Information:

- Calories: 300
- Protein: 15g
- Fat: 14g
- Carbs: 35g
- Fiber: 7g

Almond Butter and Banana Oatmeal

Ingredients:

- 1/2 cup oats
- 1 cup almond milk
- 1 banana, sliced
- 1 tablespoon almond butter
- Cinnamon, to taste

Instructions:

1. Cook oats in almond milk according to package instructions.
2. Stir in sliced banana and almond butter.

3. Sprinkle with cinnamon before serving.

Nutritional Information:

- Calories: 350
- Protein: 10g
- Fat: 15g
- Carbs: 50g
- Fiber: 7g

Mediterranean Veggie Scramble

Ingredients:

- 3 eggs
- 1/4 cup chopped bell peppers
- 1/4 cup chopped tomatoes
- 1/4 cup spinach
- 1 tablespoon olive oil
- Feta cheese, to taste
- Salt and pepper, to taste

Instructions:

1. Beat the eggs with salt and pepper.

2. Heat olive oil in a pan, add veggies, and sauté until soft.

3. Add the eggs and cook until set. Crumble feta cheese on top before serving.

Nutritional Information:

- Calories: 320
- Protein: 20g
- Fat: 24g
- Carbs: 8g
- Fiber: 2g

Turkey and Spinach Breakfast Hash

Ingredients:

- 1/2 lb lean ground turkey
- 2 cups spinach, chopped
- 1/2 cup sweet potato, cubed
- 1/4 cup onion, chopped
- 1 tablespoon olive oil
- Salt and pepper, to taste

- 1/4 teaspoon paprika

Instructions:

1. Heat olive oil in a large skillet over medium heat. Add sweet potato and onion, cooking until softened.
2. Add ground turkey, breaking it apart with a spoon, and cook until no longer pink.
3. Stir in spinach until wilted. Season with salt, pepper, and paprika.
4. Serve hot.

Nutritional Information:

- Calories: 300
- Protein: 22g
- Fat: 15g
- Carbs: 18g
- Fiber: 3g

Chapter 4

Lunch Recipes

Turkey and Veggie Stir-Fry

Ingredients:

- 4 oz lean ground turkey
- 1 cup broccoli florets
- 1/2 bell pepper, sliced
- 1/4 onion, sliced
- 1 tablespoon soy sauce (low sodium)
- 1 teaspoon sesame oil
- 1 garlic clove, minced
- Salt and pepper, to taste

Instructions:

1. Heat sesame oil in a pan over medium heat. Add garlic and onion, sautéing until fragrant.
2. Add ground turkey, breaking it apart with a spoon, and cook until browned.

3. Add broccoli and bell pepper, and cook until vegetables are tender but crisp.

4. Stir in soy sauce, season with salt and pepper, and serve.

Nutritional Information:

- Calories: 300
- Protein: 28g
- Fat: 12g
- Carbs: 18g
- Fiber: 5g

Lentil and Vegetable Soup

Ingredients:

- 1 cup lentils, rinsed
- 4 cups vegetable broth
- 1/2 cup carrots, diced
- 1/2 cup celery, diced
- 1/4 cup onion, diced
- 1 garlic clove, minced

- 1 teaspoon olive oil

- 1 teaspoon thyme

- Salt and pepper, to taste

Instructions:

1. Heat olive oil in a large pot over medium heat. Add garlic, onion, carrots, and celery. Cook until softened.

2. Add lentils, vegetable broth, and thyme. Bring to a boil, then simmer for 25-30 minutes.

3. Season with salt and pepper to taste. Serve hot.

Nutritional Information:

- Calories: 250

- Protein: 18g

- Fat: 3g

- Carbs: 40g

- Fiber: 15g

Spinach and Goat Cheese Stuffed Chicken

Ingredients:

- 4 oz chicken breast
- 1/4 cup spinach, cooked and drained
- 1 oz goat cheese
- 1 teaspoon olive oil
- Salt and pepper, to taste
- 1/2 teaspoon garlic powder

Instructions:

1. Preheat oven to 375°F (190°C).
2. Cut a slit in the chicken breast to create a pocket. Stuff with spinach and goat cheese.
3. Season the outside with salt, pepper, and garlic powder. Drizzle with olive oil.
4. Bake for 25-30 minutes, or until chicken is cooked through.

Nutritional Information:

- Calories: 320
- Protein: 30g
- Fat: 18g
- Carbs: 4g
- Fiber: 1g

Tuna Salad on Mixed Greens

Ingredients:

- 4 oz canned tuna in water, drained
- 1 tablespoon Greek yogurt
- 1/4 avocado, diced
- 1 tablespoon red onion, minced
- 1 tablespoon lemon juice
- 1 cup mixed greens
- Salt and pepper, to taste

Instructions:

1. In a bowl, mix tuna, Greek yogurt, avocado, red onion, and lemon juice. Season with salt and pepper.

2. Serve the tuna salad over a bed of mixed greens.

Nutritional Information:

- Calories: 300
- Protein: 25g
- Fat: 15g
- Carbs: 15g
- Fiber: 5g

Chickpea and Avocado Wrap

Ingredients:

- 1/2 cup chickpeas, rinsed and drained
- 1/2 avocado, mashed
- 1/4 cup diced tomatoes
- 1/4 cup shredded lettuce
- 1 whole-grain wrap
- 1 tablespoon Greek yogurt
- Salt and pepper, to taste
- A squeeze of lemon juice

Instructions:

1. Mix chickpeas, mashed avocado, diced tomatoes, and Greek yogurt in a bowl. Season with salt, pepper, and lemon juice.
2. Lay the whole-grain wrap flat and spread the chickpea mixture evenly.
3. Top with shredded lettuce, then roll the wrap tightly.
4. Serve immediately or wrap in foil for a to-go lunch.

Nutritional Information:

- Calories: 350
- Protein: 12g
- Fat: 15g
- Carbs: 45g
- Fiber: 12g

Zucchini Noodle and Pesto Chicken

Ingredients:

- 4 oz grilled chicken breast, sliced
- 2 cups zucchini noodles (zoodles)
- 2 tablespoons pesto sauce
- 1 tablespoon pine nuts
- Salt and pepper, to taste

Instructions:

1. Toss zucchini noodles with pesto sauce until evenly coated.
2. Top with sliced grilled chicken and pine nuts.
3. Season with salt and pepper to taste. Serve immediately.

Nutritional Information:

- Calories: 300
- Protein: 28g
- Fat: 18g
- Carbs: 8g
- Fiber: 2g

Beef and Broccoli Stir-Fry

Ingredients:

- 4 oz lean beef, sliced thin
- 1 cup broccoli florets
- 1/2 bell pepper, sliced
- 1 tablespoon soy sauce (low sodium)
- 1 teaspoon sesame oil
- 1 garlic clove, minced
- Salt and pepper, to taste

Instructions:

1. Heat sesame oil in a pan over medium-high heat. Add garlic and sauté until fragrant.
2. Add sliced beef, cooking until browned.
3. Add broccoli and bell pepper, cooking until vegetables are tender.
4. Stir in soy sauce, season with salt and pepper, and serve.

Nutritional Information:

- Calories: 300
- Protein: 26g
- Fat: 16g
- Carbs: 10g
- Fiber: 3g

Salmon and Asparagus Foil Packets

Ingredients:

- 4 oz salmon fillet
- 1 cup asparagus spears, trimmed
- 1 tablespoon olive oil
- 1 tablespoon lemon juice
- Salt and pepper, to taste
- 1 teaspoon dill (optional)

Instructions:

1. Preheat oven to 400°F (200°C).
2. Place salmon and asparagus on a piece of aluminum foil. Drizzle with

olive oil and lemon juice. Season with salt, pepper, and dill.

3. Fold the foil around the salmon and asparagus to create a packet.
4. Bake for 20-25 minutes, or until salmon is cooked through.

Nutritional Information:

- Calories: 300
- Protein: 23g
- Fat: 20g
- Carbs: 5g
- Fiber: 2g

Cauliflower Rice stir-fried with Shrimp

Ingredients:

- 4 oz shrimp, peeled and deveined
- 2 cups cauliflower rice
- 1/2 cup mixed vegetables (carrots, peas, bell peppers)
- 1 tablespoon soy sauce (low sodium)

- 1 teaspoon olive oil
- 1 garlic clove, minced
- Salt and pepper, to taste

Instructions:

1. Heat olive oil in a pan over medium heat. Add garlic and sauté until fragrant.
2. Add shrimp, cooking until they turn pink and opaque.
3. Add cauliflower rice and mixed vegetables, cooking until heated through.
4. Stir in soy sauce, season with salt and pepper, and serve.

Nutritional Information:

- Calories: 250
- Protein: 25g
- Fat: 8g
- Carbs: 18g
- Fiber: 5g

Mediterranean Veggie Bowl

Ingredients:

- 1/2 cup cooked quinoa
- 1/4 cup hummus
- 1/2 cup cucumber, diced
- 1/2 cup cherry tomatoes, halved
- 1/4 cup red onion, thinly sliced
- 1/4 cup kalamata olives, pitted
- 1 oz feta cheese, crumbled
- 1 tablespoon lemon juice
- 1 teaspoon olive oil
- Salt and pepper, to taste

Instructions:

1. In a bowl, layer the cooked quinoa as the base.
2. Top with hummus, cucumber, cherry tomatoes, red onion, and kalamata olives.
3. Sprinkle crumbled feta cheese over the top.

4. Drizzle with lemon juice and olive oil. Season with salt and pepper to taste.

Nutritional Information:

- Calories: 400
- Protein: 12g
- Fat: 20g
- Carbs: 45g
- Fiber: 8g

Spicy Black Bean Taco Salad

Ingredients:

- 1/2 cup black beans, rinsed and drained
- 2 cups mixed greens (lettuce, spinach, arugula)
- 1/4 cup corn
- 1/4 avocado, diced
- 1/4 cup cherry tomatoes, halved
- 1/4 cup shredded cheese (optional)

- 1 tablespoon Greek yogurt (as dressing)
- 1 tablespoon salsa
- 1 teaspoon lime juice
- Salt and pepper, to taste
- A pinch of chili flakes (optional)

Instructions:

1. In a large bowl, combine mixed greens, black beans, corn, avocado, and cherry tomatoes.
2. In a small bowl, mix Greek yogurt, salsa, and lime juice to make the dressing.
3. Drizzle the dressing over the salad, then sprinkle with shredded cheese and chili flakes if using.
4. Season with salt and pepper to taste.

Nutritional Information:

- Calories: 350
- Protein: 15g

- Fat: 15g
- Carbs: 40g
- Fiber: 12g

Chapter 5

Dinner Recipes

Salmon with Steamed Broccoli and Sweet Potato

Ingredients:

- 1 lb salmon fillet
- 2 sweet potatoes, cubed
- 2 cups broccoli florets
- 2 tbsp olive oil
- 1 tbsp garlic powder
- Salt and pepper to taste

Instructions:

1. Preheat oven to 400°F (200°C). Line a baking sheet with parchment paper.
2. Toss sweet potatoes in 1 tablespoon of olive oil, garlic powder, salt, and pepper. Spread on the baking sheet and roast for 20 minutes.

3. Season salmon with salt and pepper, place it on the baking sheet with the sweet potatoes and return to the oven. Bake for an additional 15-20 minutes or until salmon is cooked through.

4. Steam broccoli until tender, about 5 minutes.

5. Serve the salmon with roasted sweet potatoes and steamed broccoli on the side.

Nutritional Information (per serving):

- Calories: 600
- Protein: 45g
- Fats: 25g
- Carbohydrates: 45g

Macronutrient Breakdown:

- Protein: 30%
- Fats: 38%
- Carbohydrates: 32%

Turkey and Vegetable Stir-Fry

Ingredients:

- 1 lb ground turkey
- 1 cup bell peppers, sliced
- 1 cup broccoli florets
- 1/2 cup carrots, sliced
- 2 tbsp soy sauce (low sodium)
- 1 tbsp olive oil
- 1 tsp ginger, grated
- 1 garlic clove, minced
- Salt and pepper to taste

Instructions:

1. Heat olive oil in a large pan over medium heat. Add garlic and ginger, and sauté for 1 minute.
2. Add ground turkey, breaking it apart with a spatula. Cook until browned.
3. Add bell peppers, broccoli, and carrots. Stir-fry for 5-7 minutes until vegetables are tender-crisp.

4. Stir in soy sauce and cook for another 2 minutes. Season with salt and pepper to taste.

5. Serve hot.

Nutritional Information (per serving):

- Calories: 450
- Protein: 35g
- Fats: 20g
- Carbohydrates: 25g

Macronutrient Breakdown:

- Protein: 31%
- Fats: 40%
- Carbohydrates: 29%

Beef and Asparagus Skillet

Ingredients:

- 1 lb lean beef, thinly sliced
- 2 cups asparagus, trimmed and cut into pieces
- 1 tbsp olive oil

- 2 garlic cloves, minced

- 1 tbsp soy sauce (low sodium)

- 1 tsp sesame oil

- Salt and pepper to taste

Instructions:

1. Heat olive oil in a large skillet over medium-high heat. Add garlic and sauté for 30 seconds.

2. Add beef slices and cook until browned, about 3-4 minutes.

3. Add asparagus, soy sauce, and sesame oil. Stir well and cook until asparagus is tender-crisp, about 4-5 minutes.

4. Season with salt and pepper to taste. Serve immediately.

Nutritional Information (per serving):

- Calories: 400

- Protein: 40g

- Fats: 18g

- Carbohydrates: 15g

Macronutrient Breakdown:

- Protein: 40%

- Fats: 40%

- Carbohydrates: 20%

Spicy Shrimp and Cauliflower Rice

Ingredients:

- 1 lb shrimp, peeled and deveined

- 2 cups cauliflower rice

- 1 tbsp olive oil

- 1/2 cup bell peppers, diced

- 1/4 cup onions, diced

- 2 tbsp tomato sauce

- 1 tsp chili flakes (adjust to taste)

- Salt and pepper to taste

Instructions:

1. Heat olive oil in a large pan over medium heat. Add onions and bell peppers, and sauté until soft.

2. Add shrimp and cook until they turn pink, about 2-3 minutes per side.

3. Stir in cauliflower rice, tomato sauce, and chili flakes. Cook for 5-7 minutes, until everything is heated through and flavors are blended.

4. Season with salt and pepper to taste. Serve hot.

Nutritional Information (per serving):

- Calories: 300
- Protein: 35g
- Fats: 10g
- Carbohydrates: 15g

Macronutrient Breakdown:

- Protein: 47%
- Fats: 30%
- Carbohydrates: 23%

Eggplant and Chickpea Stew

Ingredients:

- 1 large eggplant, cubed
- 1 can (15 oz) chickpeas, drained and rinsed
- 1 can (14.5 oz) diced tomatoes
- 1 onion, diced
- 2 garlic cloves, minced
- 2 tbsp olive oil
- 1 tsp cumin
- 1 tsp paprika
- Salt and pepper to taste
- Fresh cilantro for garnish

Instructions:

1. Heat olive oil in a large pot over medium heat. Add onion and garlic, and cook until soft.
2. Add eggplant, chickpeas, diced tomatoes, cumin, and paprika. Stir to combine.

3. Bring to a boil, then reduce heat to low, cover, and simmer for 20-25 minutes until eggplant is tender.

4. Season with salt and pepper to taste. Garnish with fresh cilantro before serving.

Nutritional Information (per serving):

- Calories: 350
- Protein: 12g
- Fats: 14g
- Carbohydrates: 45g

Macronutrient Breakdown:

- Protein: 14%
- Fats: 36%
- Carbohydrates: 50%

Lemon Garlic Tilapia with Spinach

Ingredients:

- 4 tilapia fillets
- 4 cups fresh spinach

- 2 tbsp olive oil

- 2 garlic cloves, minced

- 1 lemon, juiced

- Salt and pepper to taste

Instructions:

1. Preheat oven to 375°F (190°C).

2. In a large skillet, heat 1 tablespoon olive oil over medium heat. Add garlic and spinach, and sauté until spinach is wilted. Remove from heat.

3. Place tilapia fillets in a baking dish. Season with salt and pepper.

4. Drizzle lemon juice and remaining olive oil over the fillets.

5. Bake in the preheated oven for 12-15 minutes, until fish flakes easily with a fork.

6. Serve the tilapia on a bed of sautéed spinach.

Nutritional Information (per serving):

- Calories: 250
- Protein: 35g
- Fats: 10g
- Carbohydrates: 5g

Macronutrient Breakdown:

- Protein: 56%
- Fats: 36%
- Carbohydrates: 8%

Stuffed Bell Peppers with Ground Turkey and Vegetables

Ingredients:

- 4 large bell peppers, tops cut, seeds removed
- 1 lb ground turkey
- 1 cup cauliflower rice
- 1 zucchini, diced
- 1 carrot, grated
- 1 onion, diced
- 2 tbsp olive oil

- 1 tsp garlic powder
- Salt and pepper to taste

Instructions:

1. Preheat oven to 350°F (175°C).
2. In a skillet, heat olive oil over medium heat. Add onion, zucchini, and carrot, and cook until soft.
3. Add ground turkey, garlic powder, salt, and pepper. Cook until turkey is browned.
4. Stir in cauliflower rice and remove from heat.
5. Stuff the bell peppers with the turkey mixture. Place in a baking dish.
6. Bake for 25-30 minutes, until peppers are tender.
7. Serve hot.

Nutritional Information (per serving):

- Calories: 350
- Protein: 25g

- Fats: 18g

- Carbohydrates: 20g

Macronutrient Breakdown:

- Protein: 29%

- Fats: 46%

- Carbohydrates: 25%

Zucchini Noodles with Avocado Pesto

Ingredients:

- 4 medium zucchinis, spiralized

- 1 ripe avocado

- 1/2 cup fresh basil leaves

- 2 tbsp pine nuts

- 2 garlic cloves

- 2 tbsp lemon juice

- 2 tbsp olive oil

- Salt and pepper to taste

- Cherry tomatoes for garnish

Instructions:

1. In a food processor, blend avocado, basil leaves, pine nuts, garlic, lemon juice, and olive oil until smooth. Season with salt and pepper.
2. In a large pan, briefly sauté the zucchini noodles in a splash of olive oil for 1-2 minutes, just until slightly softened.
3. Remove from heat and mix the avocado pesto into the zucchini noodles until well coated.
4. Serve garnished with cherry tomatoes.

Nutritional Information (per serving):

- Calories: 300
- Protein: 6g
- Fats: 25g
- Carbohydrates: 18g

Macronutrient Breakdown:

- Protein: 8%
- Fats: 75%
- Carbohydrates: 17%

Grilled Eggplant with Tofu and Tomato Sauce

Ingredients:

- 2 large eggplants, sliced into 1/2-inch rounds
- 1 lb tofu, pressed and cut into cubes
- 2 cups tomato sauce
- 2 tbsp olive oil
- 1 tsp dried oregano
- 1 tsp dried basil
- Salt and pepper to taste
- Fresh basil for garnish

Instructions:

1. Preheat the grill to medium-high heat.

2. Brush eggplant slices with olive oil and season with salt, pepper, oregano, and basil.

3. Grill eggplant slices for 4-5 minutes per side, until tender and grill marks appear.

4. In a pan, heat tomato sauce and add tofu cubes. Simmer for 5-7 minutes until heated through.

5. Serve grilled eggplant topped with tofu and tomato sauce. Garnish with fresh basil.

Nutritional Information (per serving):

- Calories: 350
- Protein: 18g
- Fats: 20g
- Carbohydrates: 25g

Macronutrient Breakdown:

- Protein: 21%

- Fats: 51%
- Carbohydrates: 28%

Baked Cod with Lemon and Dill

Ingredients:

- 4 cod fillets
- 2 lemons, sliced
- 2 tbsp olive oil
- 1 tsp dried dill
- Salt and pepper to taste

Instructions:

1. Preheat oven to 400°F (200°C).
2. Place cod fillets in a baking dish. Season with salt, pepper, and dill.
3. Drizzle with olive oil and top with lemon slices.
4. Bake for 12-15 minutes, until fish is opaque and flakes easily.
5. Serve immediately, garnished with additional lemon slices if desired.

Nutritional Information (per serving):

- Calories: 200
- Protein: 30g
- Fats: 8g
- Carbohydrates: 3g

Macronutrient Breakdown:

- Protein: 60%
- Fats: 36%
- Carbohydrates: 4%

Spiced Lentil Soup

Ingredients:

- 1 cup lentils, rinsed
- 1 onion, diced
- 2 carrots, diced
- 2 celery stalks, diced
- 2 garlic cloves, minced
- 1 tsp cumin
- 1 tsp coriander
- 4 cups vegetable broth

- 2 tbsp olive oil
- Salt and pepper to taste

Instructions:

1. Heat olive oil in a large pot over medium heat. Add onion, carrots, celery, and garlic. Cook until softened.
2. Add lentils, cumin, coriander, and vegetable broth. Bring to a boil.
3. Reduce heat and simmer for 25-30 minutes, until lentils are tender.
4. Season with salt and pepper to taste. Serve hot.

Nutritional Information (per serving):

- Calories: 250
- Protein: 15g
- Fats: 7g
- Carbohydrates: 35g

Macronutrient Breakdown:

- Protein: 24%

- Fats: 25%
- Carbohydrates: 51%

Chapter 6

Snacks and Sides

Avocado and Egg Salad

Ingredients:

- 2 hard-boiled eggs, chopped
- 1 ripe avocado, peeled and mashed
- 1 tablespoon lemon juice
- Salt and pepper to taste
- A pinch of paprika

Instructions:

1. In a bowl, mix the chopped hard-boiled eggs with the mashed avocado.
2. Add lemon juice, salt, pepper, and paprika. Mix well until combined.
3. Serve chilled as a side or a snack.

Nutritional Information (per serving):

- Calories: 300
- Protein: 12g

- Fats: 25g
- Carbohydrates: 8g

Macronutrient Breakdown:

- Protein: 16%
- Fats: 75%
- Carbohydrates: 9%

Cucumber and Hummus Bites

Ingredients:

- 1 large cucumber, sliced into rounds
- 1 cup hummus

Instructions:

1. Spread hummus on each cucumber round.
2. Serve immediately or chill before serving.

Nutritional Information (per serving):

- Calories: 150
- Protein: 6g
- Fats: 9g

- Carbohydrates: 13g

Macronutrient Breakdown:

- Protein: 16%

- Fats: 54%

- Carbohydrates: 30%

Kale Chips

Ingredients:

- 1 bunch kale, washed and dried

- 1 tablespoon olive oil

- Salt to taste

Instructions:

1. Preheat oven to 300°F (150°C).

2. Remove the kale stems and tear the leaves into bite-sized pieces.

3. Toss kale with olive oil and salt.

4. Spread on a baking sheet in a single layer.

5. Bake for 10-15 minutes until crispy.

6. Let cool before serving.

Nutritional Information (per serving):

- Calories: 100
- Protein: 3g
- Fats: 7g
- Carbohydrates: 7g

Macronutrient Breakdown:

- Protein: 12%
- Fats: 63%
- Carbohydrates: 25%

Almond Butter Celery Sticks

Ingredients:

- 3 celery stalks, cut into 3-inch pieces
- 2 tablespoons almond butter

Instructions:

1. Fill each celery piece with almond butter.
2. Serve immediately or chill before serving.

Nutritional Information (per serving):

- Calories: 150
- Protein: 4g
- Fats: 12g
- Carbohydrates: 8g

Macronutrient Breakdown:

- Protein: 11%
- Fats: 72%
- Carbohydrates: 17%

Roasted Chickpeas

Ingredients:

- 1 can (15 oz) chickpeas, drained, rinsed, and dried
- 1 tablespoon olive oil
- 1/2 teaspoon smoked paprika
- Salt to taste

Instructions:

1. Preheat oven to 400°F (200°C).
2. Toss chickpeas with olive oil, smoked paprika, and salt.

3. Spread on a baking sheet in a single
    layer.

4. Roast for 20-30 minutes until crispy,
    shaking the pan halfway through.

5. Let cool before serving.

Nutritional Information (per serving):

- Calories: 120

- Protein: 6g

- Fats: 5g

- Carbohydrates: 15g

Macronutrient Breakdown:

- Protein: 20%

- Fats: 38%

- Carbohydrates: 42%

Baked Zucchini Fries

Ingredients:

- 2 zucchinis, cut into fries

- 1/4 cup almond flour

- 1 egg, beaten

- 1/2 teaspoon garlic powder
- Salt and pepper to taste

Instructions:

1. Preheat oven to 425°F (220°C).
2. Dip zucchini fries in the beaten egg, then dredge in a mixture of almond flour, garlic powder, salt, and pepper.
3. Place on a baking sheet lined with parchment paper.
4. Bake for 20-25 minutes, flipping halfway through, until crispy and golden.
5. Serve immediately.

Nutritional Information (per serving):

- Calories: 100
- Protein: 6g
- Fats: 7g
- Carbohydrates: 6g

Macronutrient Breakdown:

- Protein: 24%

- Fats: 63%
- Carbohydrates: 13%

Cauliflower Rice Pilaf

Ingredients:

- 1 head cauliflower, riced
- 1 tablespoon olive oil
- 1/4 cup onions, diced
- 1/4 cup carrots, diced
- 1/4 cup celery, diced
- 1/2 teaspoon turmeric
- Salt and pepper to taste

Instructions:

1. Heat olive oil in a skillet over medium heat.
2. Add onions, carrots, and celery. Sauté until soft.
3. Stir in cauliflower rice and turmeric. Cook for 5-7 minutes until cauliflower is tender.

4. Season with salt and pepper to taste.

5. Serve as a side dish.

Nutritional Information (per serving):

- Calories: 80
- Protein: 3g
- Fats: 4g
- Carbohydrates: 10g

Macronutrient Breakdown:

- Protein: 15%
- Fats: 45%
- Carbohydrates: 40%

Spinach and Feta Stuffed Mushrooms

Ingredients:

- 12 large mushrooms, stems removed
- 1 cup spinach, chopped
- 1/2 cup feta cheese, crumbled
- 1 tablespoon olive oil
- Salt and pepper to taste

Instructions:

1. Preheat oven to 375°F (190°C).
2. Sauté spinach in olive oil until wilted. Let cool.
3. Mix spinach with feta cheese. Season with salt and pepper.
4. Stuff each mushroom cap with the spinach and feta mixture.
5. Bake for 15-20 minutes until mushrooms are tender.
6. Serve warm.

Nutritional Information (per serving):

- Calories: 50
- Protein: 4g
- Fats: 3g
- Carbohydrates: 2g

Macronutrient Breakdown:

- Protein: 32%
- Fats: 54%
- Carbohydrates: 14%

Smoked Salmon and Cream Cheese Cucumber Bites

Ingredients:

- 1 large cucumber, sliced into rounds
- 4 oz smoked salmon, cut into bite-sized pieces
- 1/4 cup cream cheese, softened
- Dill for garnish

Instructions:

1. Spread a small amount of cream cheese on each cucumber round.
2. Top with a piece of smoked salmon.
3. Garnish with dill.
4. Serve chilled.

Nutritional Information (per serving):

- Calories: 70
- Protein: 5g
- Fats: 5g
- Carbohydrates: 2g

Macronutrient Breakdown:

- Protein: 29%
- Fats: 64%
- Carbohydrates: 7%

Pumpkin Seeds with Tamari

Ingredients:

- 1 cup raw pumpkin seeds
- 2 tablespoons tamari or soy sauce

Instructions:

1. Preheat oven to 350°F (175°C).
2. In a bowl, toss the pumpkin seeds with tamari until evenly coated.
3. Spread the seeds on a baking sheet in a single layer.
4. Bake for 10-15 minutes, stirring occasionally, until roasted.
5. Let cool before serving.

Nutritional Information (per serving):

- Calories: 180

- Protein: 9g

- Fats: 15g

- Carbohydrates: 4g

Macronutrient Breakdown:

- Protein: 20%

- Fats: 75%

- Carbohydrates: 5%

Stuffed Mini Bell Peppers

Ingredients:

- 12 mini bell peppers, halved and seeded

- 1 cup ricotta cheese

- 1/4 cup parmesan cheese, grated

- 1 tablespoon fresh basil, chopped

- Salt and pepper to taste

Instructions:

1. Preheat oven to 375°F (190°C).

2. In a bowl, mix ricotta, parmesan, basil, salt, and pepper.

3. Fill each bell pepper half with the cheese mixture.
4. Place on a baking sheet and bake for 15-20 minutes until peppers are tender and the filling is heated through.
5. Serve warm.

Nutritional Information (per serving):

- Calories: 100
- Protein: 7g
- Fats: 6g
- Carbohydrates: 5g

Macronutrient Breakdown:

- Protein: 28%
- Fats: 54%
- Carbohydrates: 18%

Coconut Yogurt and Berry Parfait

Ingredients:

- 1 cup unsweetened coconut yogurt

- 1/2 cup mixed berries (strawberries, blueberries, raspberries)
- 1 tablespoon chia seeds
- 1 tablespoon shredded coconut, for garnish

Instructions:

1. In a serving glass, layer half of the coconut yogurt at the bottom.
2. Add a layer of mixed berries over the yogurt.
3. Sprinkle chia seeds over the berries.
4. Add another layer of coconut yogurt, then top with the remaining berries.
5. Garnish with shredded coconut.
6. Serve immediately or refrigerate until ready to serve.

Nutritional Information (per serving):

- Calories: 250
- Protein: 6g
- Fats: 15g

- Carbohydrates: 25g

Macronutrient Breakdown:

- Protein: 10%
- Fats: 54%
- Carbohydrates: 36%

Chapter 7

Desserts and Treats

Berry Chia Pudding

Ingredients:

- 1/4 cup chia seeds
- 1 cup unsweetened almond milk
- 1/2 cup mixed berries
- 1 tbsp monk fruit sweetener

Instructions:

1. Mix chia seeds with almond milk and sweetener. Let sit for 15 minutes.
2. Stir in berries and refrigerate overnight.

Nutritional Information:

- Carbs: 40%
- Protein: 10%
- Fat: 50%

Almond Flour Lemon Bars

Ingredients:

- 2 cups almond flour
- 1/2 cup coconut oil, melted
- 1/4 cup monk fruit sweetener
- 4 eggs
- Juice and zest from 2 lemons

Instructions:

1. Mix almond flour, coconut oil, and sweetener for the crust. Press into a pan and bake at 350°F for 15 minutes.
2. Whisk eggs, lemon juice, and zest, pour over the crust, and bake for 20 minutes.

Nutritional Information:

- Carbs: 20%
- Protein: 15%
- Fat: 65%

Coconut Yogurt Parfait

Ingredients:

- 1 cup unsweetened coconut yogurt
- 1/4 cup granola (low carb)
- 1/2 cup raspberries

Instructions:

1. Layer yogurt, granola, and raspberries in a glass.

Nutritional Information:

- Carbs: 30%
- Protein: 10%
- Fat: 60%

Protein-Packed Chocolate Shake

Ingredients:

- 1 scoop of chocolate protein powder
- 1 cup unsweetened almond milk
- 1 tbsp almond butter
- Ice cubes

Instructions:

1. Blend all ingredients until smooth.

Nutritional Information:

- Carbs: 20%

- Protein: 60%

- Fat: 20%

Keto Blueberry Muffins

Ingredients:

- 2 cups almond flour

- 3 eggs

- 1/4 cup coconut oil, melted

- 1/2 cup erythritol

- 1 cup blueberries

Instructions:

1. Mix almond flour, eggs, coconut oil, and erythritol. Fold in blueberries.

2. Bake at 350°F for 25 minutes.

Nutritional Information:

- Carbs: 15%

- Protein: 15%

- Fat: 70%

Cinnamon Flaxseed Crackers

Ingredients:

- 1 cup flaxseed meal

- 1 tsp cinnamon

- 1/2 cup water

- Pinch of salt

Instructions:

1. Mix all ingredients and spread thinly on a baking sheet.

2. Bake at 350°F until crisp.

Nutritional Information:

- Carbs: 10%

- Protein: 20%

- Fat: 70%

Almond Butter Cups

Ingredients:

- 1 cup dark chocolate (at least 85% cocoa)
- 1/2 cup almond butter
- 1 tbsp coconut oil

Instructions:

1. Melt chocolate and coconut oil. Pour a layer into muffin cups, and freeze until set.
2. Add almond butter, top with more chocolate, and freeze.

Nutritional Information:

- Carbs: 20%
- Protein: 10%
- Fat: 70%

Strawberry Gelatin Squares

Ingredients:

- 2 cups fresh strawberries
- 1/4 cup water
- 2 tbsp gelatin powder
- 1 tbsp monk fruit sweetener

Instructions:

1. Blend strawberries and water, heat slightly, and mix in gelatin and sweetener.
2. Pour into a mold and refrigerate until set.

Nutritional Information:

- Carbs: 30%
- Protein: 20%
- Fat: 50%

Pumpkin Seed Brittle

Ingredients:

- 1 cup pumpkin seeds

- 1/2 cup monk fruit sweetener

- 1/4 cup water

Instructions:

1. Heat sweetener and water until caramelized, stir in pumpkin seeds, and spread on a baking sheet to cool.

Nutritional Information:

- Carbs: 10%

- Protein: 30%

- Fat: 60%

Vanilla Protein Bars

Ingredients:

- 2 cups protein powder (vanilla)

- 1/2 cup almond milk

- 1/4 cup almond butter

- 1 tsp vanilla extract

Instructions:

1. Mix all ingredients, press into a pan, and refrigerate until firm.

Nutritional Information:

- Carbs: 20%
- Protein: 50%
- Fat: 30%

Cocoa-Nut Energy Balls

Ingredients:
- 1 cup walnuts
- 1/2 cup shredded coconut
- 1/4 cup cocoa powder
- 1/4 cup coconut oil
- 1 tbsp monk fruit sweetener

Instructions:

1. Blend all ingredients and form into balls. Refrigerate until firm.

Nutritional Information:

- Carbs: 10%

- Protein: 15%
- Fat: 75%

Chapter 8

Beverages

Green Tea Metabolism Booster

Ingredients:

- 1 bag of green tea

- 1 cup hot water
- 1 tbsp lemon juice
- 1 tsp grated ginger
- 1 tbsp honey (optional, for those not strictly avoiding sugars)

Instructions:

1. Steep green tea in hot water for 3-5 minutes.
2. Add lemon juice and grated ginger.
3. Stir in honey if using. Serve hot.

Nutritional Information:

- Carbs: 90% (if honey is used, otherwise significantly lower)

- Protein: 0%
- Fat: 10%

Keto Chocolate Smoothie

Ingredients:

- 1 scoop of chocolate protein powder
- 1 cup unsweetened almond milk
- 1 tbsp unsweetened cocoa powder
- 1 tbsp almond butter
- Ice cubes

Instructions:

1. Blend all ingredients until smooth.

Nutritional Information:

- Carbs: 10%
- Protein: 60%
- Fat: 30%

Cucumber Mint Detox Water

Ingredients:

- 1/2 cucumber, sliced

- 10 mint leaves
- 1 liter water

Instructions:

1. Combine all ingredients in a pitcher.
2. Chill for at least 1 hour before serving.

Nutritional Information:

- Carbs: 5%
- Protein: 0%
- Fat: 0%

Turmeric Ginger Tea

Ingredients:

- 1 tsp turmeric powder
- 1 tsp grated ginger
- 1 cup hot water
- 1 tbsp lemon juice

Instructions:

1. Steep turmeric and ginger in hot water for 5-10 minutes.

2. Strain and add lemon juice. Serve hot.

Nutritional Information:

- Carbs: 20%
- Protein: 0%
- Fat: 10%

Berry Protein Shake

Ingredients:

- 1 scoop vanilla protein powder
- 1 cup mixed berries (frozen)
- 1 cup unsweetened almond milk
- Ice cubes

Instructions:

1. Blend all ingredients until smooth.

Nutritional Information:

- Carbs: 30%
- Protein: 50%
- Fat: 20%

Lemon Ginger Zinger Shot

Ingredients:

- 1/4 cup fresh lemon juice
- 1-inch ginger root, juiced
- 1/4 tsp cayenne pepper

Instructions:

1. Mix lemon juice, ginger juice, and cayenne pepper.
2. Consume immediately.

Nutritional Information:

- Carbs: 90%
- Protein: 0%
- Fat: 10%

Coconut Water Electrolyte Drink

Ingredients:

- 1 cup coconut water
- 1/2 cup water
- 1 tbsp lemon juice
- A pinch of sea salt

Instructions:

1. Combine all ingredients and stir well.

Nutritional Information:

- Carbs: 25%
- Protein: 0%
- Fat: 0%

Spicy Tomato Juice

Ingredients:

- 1 cup tomato juice (low sodium)
- 1/2 tsp Worcestershire sauce
- 1/2 tsp hot sauce
- 1/2 tsp lemon juice
- Pinch of salt and pepper

Instructions:

1. Combine all ingredients and stir well. Serve chilled.

Nutritional Information:

- Carbs: 90%
- Protein: 5%

- Fat: 5%

Matcha Latte

Ingredients:

- 1 tsp matcha powder
- 1 cup unsweetened almond milk
- 1 tsp honey (optional)

Instructions:

1. Dissolve matcha in a small amount of hot water.
2. Heat almond milk and add to matcha. Sweeten with honey if desired.

Nutritional Information:

- Carbs: 30% (with honey) or 20% (without honey)
- Protein: 20%
- Fat: 50%

Golden Milk

Ingredients:

- 1 cup almond milk
- 1 tsp turmeric powder
- 1/2 tsp cinnamon
- 1/4 tsp ginger powder
- 1 tbsp honey (optional)

Instructions:

1. Heat almond milk and whisk in turmeric, cinnamon, and ginger.
2. Sweeten with honey if desired. Serve warm.

Nutritional Information:

- Carbs: 30% (with honey) or 20% (without honey)
- Protein: 0%
- Fat: 70%

Aloe Vera Refresh Drink

Ingredients:

- 1 cup aloe vera juice
- 1 cup cucumber, chopped
- 1 tbsp lemon juice
- 1 tbsp honey (optional)

Instructions:

1. Blend aloe vera juice, cucumber, and lemon juice until smooth.
2. Sweeten with honey if desired.

Nutritional Information:

- Carbs: 80% (with honey) or 70% (without honey)
- Protein: 0%
- Fat: 20%

Avocado Smoothie

Ingredients:

- 1 ripe avocado
- 1 cup unsweetened almond milk

- 1 tbsp lemon juice
- 1 tbsp honey (optional)
- Ice cubes

Instructions:

1. Blend all ingredients until smooth.

Nutritional Information:

- Carbs: 30% (with honey) or 20% (without honey)
- Protein: 10%
- Fat: 60%

Apple Cider Vinegar Tonic

Ingredients:

- 1 tbsp apple cider vinegar
- 1 cup water
- 1 tbsp honey (optional)
- 1 tsp lemon juice

Instructions:

1. Mix apple cider vinegar, water, honey (if using), and lemon juice.

2. Drink in the morning on an empty stomach.

Nutritional Information:

- Carbs: 90% (with honey) or 80% (without honey)
- Protein: 0%
- Fat: 10%

Cinnamon Almond Milk Warmer

Ingredients:

- 1 cup unsweetened almond milk
- 1/2 tsp ground cinnamon
- 1/4 tsp vanilla extract
- 1 tsp honey (optional for those who include natural sweeteners)

Instructions:

1. Heat almond milk in a small saucepan over medium heat.
2. Stir in cinnamon and vanilla extract.

3. Sweeten with honey if using. Heat until warm but not boiling.

4. Serve immediately.

Nutritional Information:

- Carbs: 30% (with honey) or 20% (without honey)
- Protein: 0%
- Fat: 70%

Chapter 9

Supplements and Support

Recommended Supplements for Endomorphs

Endomorphs, characterized by a tendency to gain weight easily, especially in the form of fat, and a harder time losing it, may benefit from specific supplements to enhance their metabolism and support their body composition goals. However, it's crucial to remember that supplements should complement, not replace, a nutritious diet and regular exercise.

1.	**Protein Powders (Whey, Pea, Hemp):** Protein is essential for muscle repair, growth, and maintaining a feeling of fullness. Protein supplements can help ensure endomorphs meet their protein requirements, which can aid in fat loss and muscle maintenance.

2.   **Omega-3 Fatty Acids**: Found in fish oil or algal oil supplements, omega-3s can help improve body composition by enhancing fat loss and reducing inflammation, which is often higher in individuals with excess body fat.

3.   **Green Tea Extract**: Known for its metabolism-boosting properties, green tea extract can enhance fat oxidation and contribute to a slight increase in calorie burning throughout the day.

4.   **Conjugated Linoleic Acid (CLA)**: CLA has been shown to help reduce body fat in some studies by enhancing fat metabolism and inhibiting fat production.

5.   **Chromium Picolinate**: This supplement may help improve insulin sensitivity and glucose metabolism, which can be beneficial for weight management.

6. **Soluble Fiber Supplements (Glucomannan)**: Soluble fiber can help increase feelings of fullness, decrease appetite, and improve gut health, aiding in weight management.

Importance of Hydration

Hydration plays a crucial role in maintaining optimal metabolic function and overall health. For endomorphs, staying adequately hydrated is essential for several reasons:

- **Enhanced Metabolism**: Proper hydration can slightly increase the rate at which your body burns calories. Even mild dehydration can slow down metabolism.

- **Appetite Regulation**: Sometimes, the body can confuse signals of dehydration with hunger. Staying hydrated can help regulate appetite and prevent overeating.

- **Improved Exercise Performance**: Adequate hydration is vital for maintaining energy levels and performance during exercise, which is crucial for endomorphs focusing on weight management and muscle toning.
- **Detoxification and Digestion**: Water helps to flush out toxins, maintain healthy digestion, and prevent constipation, supporting overall health and weight management efforts.

Supporting Metabolism Naturally

Endomorphs can adopt several strategies to support and enhance their metabolism naturally, beyond diet and exercise:

1. **Regular Physical Activity**: Incorporating both cardio and strength training can increase muscle mass, which

in turn can boost metabolic rate since muscle burns more calories than fat.

2.   **Eating Protein-Rich Foods**: Protein has a higher thermic effect than fats and carbohydrates, meaning your body uses more energy to digest it, which can boost metabolism.

3.   **Managing Stress**: High levels of cortisol, the stress hormone, can lead to weight gain, especially around the midsection. Practices such as meditation, yoga, and adequate sleep can help manage stress.

4.   **Timing Meals**: Eating at regular intervals can help maintain steady blood sugar levels, preventing spikes and crashes that can lead to overeating. Some find eating smaller, more frequent meals beneficial, though individual responses may vary.

5.   **Spicy Foods**: Capsaicin, found in chili peppers, can provide a temporary boost in metabolism and increase fat burning.

6.   **Getting Enough Sleep**: Lack of sleep can disrupt hormones that regulate appetite, leading to increased hunger and calorie intake.

Incorporating these supplements and practices can support endomorphs in achieving a more balanced metabolism and healthier body composition.

Chapter 10

Best Workouts Exercise for Endomorphs

Resistance Training Workout Plan:

Warm-Up (5-10 minutes):

- Perform a dynamic warm-up to prepare your muscles and joints for exercise.
- Include movements such as arm circles, leg swings, bodyweight squats, lunges, and shoulder rolls.
- Aim to elevate your heart rate and increase blood flow to the muscles.

Main Workout (30-45 minutes):

1. **Exercise Selection**: Choose 6-8 exercises targeting major muscle groups (legs, back, chest, shoulders, arms, and core).

2. **Sets and Reps**: Perform 2-3 sets of each exercise with 8-12 repetitions per set.

3. **Rest Periods**: Rest for 60-90 seconds between sets to allow for adequate recovery.

4. **Progressive Overload**: Increase the weight or resistance when you can comfortably complete all sets and reps with good form.

Sample Workout:

- Squats (Legs)
- Push-ups (Chest)
- Bent-over Rows (Back)
- Shoulder Press (Shoulders)
- Bicep Curls (Arms)
- Tricep Dips (Arms)
- Planks (Core)
- Russian Twists (Core)

Cool Down and Stretching (5-10 minutes):

- Perform static stretches targeting major muscle groups to improve flexibility and reduce muscle tension.

- Hold each stretch for 15-30 seconds, focusing on breathing deeply and relaxing into the stretch.

- Focus on areas that were worked during the workout, such as hamstrings, quadriceps, chest, back, shoulders, and arms.

Cardiovascular Exercise plan workout plan

Warm-Up (5-10 minutes):

- Begin with a 5-10 minute dynamic warm-up to prepare your body for cardiovascular activity.

- Include movements such as jogging in place, jumping jacks, arm swings, leg swings, and hip circles.

- Gradually increase your heart rate and blood flow to the muscles.

Main Cardiovascular Workout (20-30 minutes):

1. **Choose Your Activity**: Select a cardiovascular exercise that you enjoy and can sustain for the duration of the workout. Options include:
   - Brisk walking or power walking
   - Running or jogging
   - Cycling (outdoors or stationary bike)
   - Swimming
   - Dancing
   - Jumping rope
   - Rowing
   - Stair climbing
2. **Set Your Intensity**: Determine your intensity level based on your fitness level and goals. Beginners may start

with moderate intensity (where you can talk but not sing), while more advanced individuals can aim for higher intensity (where talking becomes challenging).

3. **Duration**: Aim for 20-30 minutes of continuous cardiovascular exercise. Start with a duration that feels comfortable and gradually increase over time as your fitness improves.

4. **Interval Training (Optional)**: For added variety and intensity, incorporate interval training into your cardiovascular workout. Alternate between periods of higher intensity (e.g., faster pace or higher resistance) and lower intensity (e.g., slower pace or lower resistance) throughout the workout.

Cool Down and Stretching (5-10 minutes):

- After completing the main cardiovascular workout, cool down with 5-10 minutes of low-intensity activity such as walking or gentle cycling.
- Follow the cool down with static stretching to improve flexibility and reduce muscle tension.
- Focus on stretching major muscle groups, including hamstrings, quadriceps, calves, chest, back, shoulders, and arms.
- Hold each stretch for 15-30 seconds, breathing deeply and relaxing into the stretch.

Circuit Training workout plan:

Warm-Up (5-10 minutes):

- Begin with a dynamic warm-up to prepare your body for exercise and increase blood flow to the muscles.
- Include movements such as arm circles, leg swings, bodyweight squats, lunges, and jogging in place.
- Gradually increase the intensity to elevate your heart rate and warm up your muscles.

Circuit Training Circuit (Repeat 3-4 Times):

Perform each exercise for the specified duration or number of repetitions, moving from one exercise to the next with minimal rest in between. Once you complete all exercises in the circuit, rest for 1-2 minutes, then repeat the circuit for a total of 3-4 rounds.

1. **Bodyweight Squats (45 seconds)**:

   - Stand with feet shoulder-width apart, chest up, and core engaged.
   - Lower your body by bending your knees and pushing your hips back as if sitting in a chair.
   - Keep your weight on your heels and lower until your thighs are parallel to the ground.
   - Push through your heels to return to the starting position.

2. **Push-Ups (10-12 repetitions)**:

   - Start in a high plank position with hands shoulder-width apart and core engaged.
   - Lower your body by bending your elbows until your chest nearly touches the ground.

- Keep your body in a straight line from head to heels.
- Push through your palms to return to the starting position.

3. **Jumping Jacks (45 seconds)**:
   - Stand with feet together and arms at your sides.
   - Jump your feet out to the sides while simultaneously raising your arms overhead.
   - Jump back to the starting position with feet together and arms at your sides.
   - Repeat in a fluid motion.

4. **Dumbbell Rows (10-12 repetitions per arm)**:
   - Hold a dumbbell in one hand, hinge forward at the hips, and brace your opposite hand on a

bench or sturdy surface for support.

- Pull the dumbbell towards your hip, keeping your elbow close to your body and squeezing your shoulder blade.

- Lower the dumbbell with control and repeat on the opposite side.

5. **Mountain Climbers (45 seconds)**:

- Start in a high plank position with wrists under shoulders and core engaged.

- Drive one knee towards your chest while keeping the other leg extended.

- Quickly switch legs, alternating knees in a running motion.

- Keep your hips low and core tight throughout the movement.

6. **Plank Hold (30-45 seconds)**:

    - Start in a high plank position with wrists under shoulders and core engaged.

    - Keep your body in a straight line from head to heels, avoiding sagging or arching.

    - Hold the position, focusing on maintaining tension in your core and breathing rhythmically.

Cool Down and Stretching (5-10 minutes):

- After completing the circuit training circuit, cool down with 5-10 minutes of low-intensity activity such as walking or gentle cycling.

- Follow the cool down with static stretching to improve flexibility and reduce muscle tension.
- Focus on stretching major muscle groups, holding each stretch for 15-30 seconds, and breathing deeply.

Flexibility and Mobility Workout Plan:

Warm-Up (5-10 minutes):

- Start with 5-10 minutes of light aerobic activity such as walking, jogging, or cycling to increase blood flow to the muscles and prepare the body for stretching.

Dynamic Stretching (5-10 minutes):

- Perform dynamic stretches that move your muscles and joints through a full range of motion.

- Include movements such as arm circles, leg swings, hip circles, shoulder rolls, and trunk twists.
- Focus on controlled movements and gradually increase the intensity of the stretches as your muscles warm up.

Static Stretching (10-15 minutes):

- Hold each static stretch for 15-30 seconds, focusing on the major muscle groups used during exercise.
- Breathe deeply and relax into each stretch, avoiding any bouncing or jerking movements.
- Focus on areas such as hamstrings, quadriceps, calves, hip flexors, chest, back, shoulders, and arms.
- Use props such as yoga blocks or straps to assist with stretching and improve flexibility.

Foam Rolling or Self-Myofascial Release (5-10 minutes):

- Use a foam roller or massage ball to target tight or sore muscles and release tension in the fascia (connective tissue).
- Roll slowly and deliberately over areas of tightness, pausing on any tender spots for 20-30 seconds to allow the tissue to release.
- Focus on areas such as the calves, hamstrings, quadriceps, IT band, glutes, upper back, and shoulders.
- Adjust the pressure by shifting your body weight and breathing deeply to facilitate relaxation.

Mobility Exercises (10-15 minutes):

- Perform mobility exercises to improve joint mobility and enhance movement quality.

- Include movements such as hip circles, shoulder circles, thoracic spine rotations, wrist circles, ankle circles, and neck stretches.
- Focus on controlled, deliberate movements, exploring your full range of motion while maintaining proper alignment.
- Pay attention to areas of stiffness or restriction and work on gently mobilizing those joints.

Cool Down (5-10 minutes):

- Finish with 5-10 minutes of gentle stretching and deep breathing to promote relaxation and reduce muscle tension.
- Focus on slow, rhythmic movements and deep diaphragmatic breathing to help calm the nervous system and aid in recovery.

Consistency and Progression:

Regardless of the specific workouts chosen, consistency and progression are key for endomorphs to see results. Gradually increase the intensity, duration, or resistance of your workouts over time to continue challenging your body and avoiding plateaus. Additionally, prioritize recovery with adequate rest, hydration, and nutrition to support your fitness journey. Remember, the best workout for you is one that you enjoy and can sustain long-term. Experiment with different types of exercises and find what works best for your body and lifestyle. Consulting with a certified personal trainer or fitness professional can also help tailor a workout plan specifically to your needs and goals as an endomorph.

Incorporating Movement into Your Routine

Here are some effective strategies for integrating more physical activity into your daily life:

1. Set Realistic Goals:

Start by setting achievable goals that align with your current fitness level and lifestyle. Whether it's walking for 30 minutes a day, taking the stairs instead of the elevator, or doing a quick workout at home, establishing realistic objectives will help you stay motivated and consistent.

2. Find Activities You Enjoy:

Choose activities that you genuinely enjoy, as you're more likely to stick with them long-term. Whether it's dancing, hiking, swimming, or playing a sport, make movement enjoyable. Experiment with different activities until you find what resonates with you.

3. Schedule Physical Activity:

Treat exercise like any other appointment by scheduling it into your daily routine. Set aside dedicated time for physical activity, whether it's in the morning before work, during your lunch break, or in the evening after dinner. Consistency is key, so aim for at least 30 minutes of moderate-intensity exercise most days of the week.

4. Break It Up:

If finding time for a single, continuous workout is challenging, break it up into shorter bouts of activity throughout the day. Take three 10-minute walks, do a quick bodyweight workout during commercial breaks, or incorporate stretching sessions into your breaks at work.

5. Make It Social:

Exercise with friends, family, or coworkers to make it more enjoyable and hold yourself accountable. Join a sports team, participate in group fitness classes, or simply go for walks together. Not only does socializing move more fun, but it also provides additional motivation and support.

6. Multitask:

Look for opportunities to incorporate movement into your daily tasks and errands. Walk or bike instead of driving whenever possible, do household chores like vacuuming or gardening, or take the opportunity to stretch while watching TV or talking on the phone.

7. Be Mindful:

Practice mindfulness during every day activities by focusing on your body and movement. Pay attention to your posture, engage your muscles, and move with intention. This mindfulness can help improve your movement patterns, reduce the risk of injury, and enhance the overall benefits of physical activity.

8. Track Your Progress:

Keep track of your physical activity to monitor your progress and celebrate your achievements. Use a fitness tracker, journal, or smartphone app to record your workouts, steps taken, or active minutes. Seeing your progress over time can be incredibly motivating and help you stay committed to your fitness goals.

Chapter 11

Conclusion

In conclusion, the Metabolic Reset Diet tailored specifically for endomorphs presents a comprehensive and profitable solution for those seeking to optimize their metabolism, achieve sustainable weight loss, and attain overall well-being. Through a strategic blend of nutritional principles, lifestyle adjustments, and targeted dietary strategies, this specialized diet plan offers a pathway to transformative results and long-term success.

By addressing the unique metabolic characteristics of endomorphs, including a propensity for storing excess fat and a slower metabolic rate, the Metabolic Reset Diet provides a tailored approach that targets underlying metabolic imbalances and promotes positive metabolic adaptations. Through the careful selection of nutrient-dense foods, portion control, and balanced macronutrient distribution, individuals can effectively regulate blood sugar levels, optimize energy production, and enhance metabolic efficiency.

Moreover, the Metabolic Reset Diet emphasizes the importance of incorporating regular physical activity, including both cardiovascular exercise and strength training, to further amplify metabolic benefits, stimulate fat loss, and support overall health. By combining dietary modifications with a consistent exercise regimen, individuals can maximize their metabolic potential, accelerate weight loss, and improve body composition.

Beyond the physical benefits, the Metabolic Reset Diet offers a holistic approach to wellness that encompasses the mental, emotional, and social aspects of health. By fostering a positive relationship with food, promoting mindful eating habits, and prioritizing self-care practices, individuals can cultivate a sustainable lifestyle that nourishes both body and mind.

Furthermore, the profitability of the Metabolic Reset Diet extends beyond individual health outcomes to encompass broader societal benefits. As individuals experience improvements in metabolic health, they may also reduce their risk of chronic diseases such as obesity, diabetes, and cardiovascular disease, resulting in decreased healthcare costs and improved quality of life for both individuals and society as a whole.

In essence, the Metabolic Reset Diet for endomorphs represents a profitable investment in long-term health and vitality. By embracing this specialized dietary approach, individuals can unlock their metabolic potential, achieve their weight loss goals, and embark on a journey towards lasting transformation.

BONUS

<u>Customized Metabolic Reset Food list</u>

Proteins

- **Lean Meats**: Chicken breast, turkey, lean beef cuts, and pork loin.
- **Fish and Seafood**: Salmon, mackerel, sardines, trout, shrimp, and scallops.
- **Eggs**: Whole eggs and egg whites.
- **Plant-Based Proteins**: Lentils, chickpeas, black beans, kidney beans, and tofu.

Vegetables (Non-Starchy)

- **Leafy Greens**: Spinach, kale, collard greens, and Swiss chard.
- **Cruciferous Vegetables**: Broccoli, cauliflower, Brussels sprouts, and cabbage.

- **Other Vegetables**: Asparagus, zucchini, bell peppers, and cucumbers.

Low-Glycemic Fruits

- **Berries**: Strawberries, blueberries, raspberries, and blackberries.
- **Citrus Fruits**: Oranges, lemons, limes, and grapefruits.
- **Apples and Pears**: Opt for whole fruits rather than juices for added fiber.

Whole Grains and Complex Carbohydrates

- **Oats**: Steel-cut or old-fashioned oats.
- **Quinoa**: A complete protein and a good source of fiber.
- **Brown Rice and Wild Rice**: More fiber and nutrients than white rice.
- **Sweet Potatoes**: A better option than regular potatoes due to their lower GI.

Healthy Fats

- **Avocados**: Rich in monounsaturated fats and fiber.
- **Nuts and Seeds**: Almonds, walnuts, chia seeds, and flaxseeds.
- **Olive Oil**: Use in cooking or as a salad dressing.
- **Fatty Fish**: Provides omega-3 fatty acids.

Dairy or Dairy Alternatives

- **Greek Yogurt**: Opt for low-fat or full-fat versions without added sugar.
- **Cottage Cheese**: A good source of protein.
- **Almond Milk**: Unsweetened varieties to avoid added sugars.

Beverages

- **Water**: Aim for at least 8 glasses a day.
- **Green Tea**: Can help boost metabolism.

- **Black Coffee**: In moderation, without added sugar or cream.

Spices and Herbs

- **Turmeric**: Has anti-inflammatory properties.
- **Cinnamon**: Can help manage blood sugar levels.
- **Ginger**: Good for digestion and metabolism.
- **Cayenne Pepper**: May boost metabolism.

<u>Lifestyle and Wellness Tips</u>

For endomorphs, or anyone looking to enhance their metabolism and overall wellness, adopting certain lifestyle and wellness tips can be transformative. These tips are designed to complement a balanced diet, helping to boost metabolism, manage weight, and improve overall health.

Here are some practical lifestyle and wellness tips to consider:

1. Regular Physical Activity

- **Strength Training**: Building muscle mass is crucial for endomorphs as muscle burns more calories at rest compared to fat. Aim for at least 2-3 strength training sessions per week.

- **Cardiovascular Exercise**: Incorporate HIIT (High-Intensity Interval Training) or moderate-intensity cardio exercises like brisk walking, cycling, or swimming for 150 minutes weekly to burn fat and improve heart health.

- **Consistency is Key**: Find activities you enjoy to ensure you can stick with them long-term.

2. Mindful Eating

- **Listen to Your Body**: Eat when you're hungry and stop when you're satisfied. Learn to differentiate between true hunger and emotional or habitual eating.
- **Slow Down**: Eating slowly can help you better recognize your body's satiety signals, reducing the likelihood of overeating.

3. Hydration

- **Water Intake**: Drink at least 8 glasses of water daily, or more if you're active or live in a hot climate. Hydration is essential for metabolism and helps reduce appetite.
- **Limit Sugary and High-Calorie Beverages**: Opt for water, herbal teas, or black coffee instead of

sugary sodas, juices, or alcoholic drinks.

4. Stress Management

- **Meditation and Yoga**: These practices can help reduce stress, which is important because high-stress levels can lead to weight gain, especially in the abdominal area.

- **Regular Relaxation**: Make time for activities that relax and rejuvenate you, whether it's reading, taking a bath, or walking in nature.

5. Quality Sleep

- **Regular Sleep Schedule**: Aim for 7-9 hours of quality sleep per night and try to go to bed and wake up at the same times every day.

- **Sleep Environment**: Ensure your bedroom is conducive to sleep—dark, quiet, and cool.

6. Positive Social Connections

- **Support Network**: Surround yourself with a supportive community, whether friends, family, or groups who share your wellness goals.
- **Social Activities**: Engage in social activities that don't revolve around food or alcohol but rather focus on shared interests or hobbies.

7. Set Realistic Goals

- **SMART Goals**: Ensure your wellness goals are Specific, Measurable, Achievable, Relevant, and Time-bound.
- **Celebrate Progress**: Recognize and celebrate your achievements, no matter how small, to stay motivated.

8. Continuous Learning

- **Stay Informed**: Keep learning about nutrition, exercise, and wellness to find what works best for your body.
- **Adapt and Adjust**: Be willing to adjust your approach as you learn what does and doesn't work for you.

9. Mindset

- **Positive Mindset**: Maintain a positive outlook and be patient with yourself. Wellness is a journey, not a destination.
- **Self-Compassion**: Treat yourself with kindness and understanding, avoiding negative self-talk or comparison with others.